Mastering ADHD: Tools for Personal and Professional Success

Preface

Thank you for purchasing this short book on mastering ADHD. I wrote this because I wish someone had given me something similar when I first realized that I had ADHD. It can be a scary feeling, but you're still the same person you've always been, you're still you. You just have a better understanding of *why* you're you now.

This was written to help people of all ages deal with ADHD, but I hope this serves as a resource for adults especially. I don't believe that adult ADHD is talked about enough. We're essentially told to tough it out. You've probably heard someone tell you that "ADHD isn't real." Or that they might have a "little ADHD themself." It used to bother me, but honestly, who cares what anyone else thinks?

Introduction

This topic is personal to me and the culmination of over 15 years of being diagnosed with ADHD, or attention-deficit/hyperactivity disorder. It's a disorder that's misunderstood, misappropriated, and hard to explain to someone who doesn't have to deal with it. I'll start with a basic overview of ADHD, then a bit about my story, and then we'll review some of my favorite strategies for managing and conquering ADHD. I recommend this book to people dealing with ADHD and people who have close relationships with people with ADHD. For simplicity's sake, I'll refer to it as ADHD, but it was also known as ADD. As far as I've been able to tell, there is no difference between the two.

Understanding ADHD

Attention Deficit Hyperactivity Disorder (ADHD) is a neurodevelopmental disorder that affects individuals across various age groups, including children, adolescents, and adults. To effectively help people manage ADHD and succeed in both their professional and personal lives, it's important to have an understanding of this condition.

Core symptoms of inattention, hyperactivity, and impulsivity characterize ADHD. Individuals with ADHD often struggle with focusing on tasks, following through with responsibilities, and controlling their impulses. These challenges can significantly impact our daily lives, from academic and work performance to relationships. I can personally attest to the struggles I've faced in my relationships and, to a degree, my professional performance.

ADHD is not a result of laziness or lack of willpower; it's a neurobiological condition with a genetic component. People with ADHD are often incorrectly labeled as "lazy", and it used to bother me when someone would call me lazy, knowing how hard I worked and continue to work on myself and what's important to me. Research suggests that imbalances in neurotransmitters, particularly dopamine and norepinephrine, play a significant role in the development of ADHD. This understanding helps us destigmatize the condition and emphasizes that people with ADHD face unique cognitive challenges.

It's important to note that ADHD is a spectrum disorder, meaning that its severity can vary among individuals. Some may primarily struggle with inattention, while others exhibit more hyperactive and impulsive behaviors. This diversity in symptom presentation underscores the need for personalized strategies and interventions.

ADHD often presents co-occurring conditions, such as anxiety and depression. I have struggled with both of these co-occurring conditions myself, unfortunately. Understanding these comorbidities is crucial, as they can exacerbate the challenges associated with ADHD. Additionally, ADHD can persist into adulthood, and many may go undiagnosed until later in life, making it essential to recognize and address the condition at any age. Someone close to me was diagnosed at 35, and I remember him telling me everything "clicked" for him once he was diagnosed. It was the first step in working on himself and seeing his progress since diagnosis has been incredible.

Furthermore, the impact of ADHD extends beyond the individual diagnosed. Family members, friends, and colleagues can also be affected, which emphasizes the importance of providing support and education to create a more inclusive and accommodating environment.

Diagnosis & Assessment

ADHD diagnosis typically involves a comprehensive evaluation considering various aspects of an individual's life. Diagnosis begins with gathering information from multiple sources, including self-reports, parents, teachers, and others close to the person. This holistic approach helps paint a complete picture of the individual's behavior and symptoms, considering different environments such as home, school, and work. These insights are essential for an accurate assessment.

A key aspect of the diagnostic process is the identification of specific ADHD symptoms. Clinicians use established criteria, such as those from the Diagnostic and Statistical Manual of Mental Disorders (DSM-5), to assess whether these symptoms are present and to what extent they interfere with daily life. ADHD assessments may also consider the presence of coexisting conditions, such as anxiety or depression, which can complicate the clinical picture. These comorbidities should be addressed as part of the assessment process to ensure comprehensive care.

A proper diagnosis often involves ruling out other medical or psychiatric conditions that may mimic ADHD symptoms. This process helps prevent misdiagnosis and ensures that individuals receive the most appropriate treatment and support. In recent years, there has been a growing recognition of adult ADHD, which can sometimes go undiagnosed. Clinicians must consider the possibility of ADHD in adults as well and assess their symptoms within the context of their daily lives and responsibilities.

The diagnostic journey may include various assessments, questionnaires, and interviews to gain a comprehensive understanding of the individual's challenges and strengths. This process helps people with ADHD receive the right interventions and support tailored to their needs. A professional diagnosis, in my experience, also helps with one's mental health. Knowing what to deal with is a lot easier than questioning why you're "different" or "lazy" or "inattentive." It's a vindicating feeling, at least it was for me.

Self-Aware or Self-Sabatoge?

I grew up with three younger brothers and two fantastic parents who worked extremely hard to give all of us a good childhood. My brothers and I were enrolled at a Catholic school from kindergarten through middle school, and we excelled academically. The difference between my brothers and me, however, was evident when parent-teacher conferences happened. I was talkative, occasionally disruptive, and needed stimulation.

Since I was able to understand the material fairly quickly, I spent a lot of time waiting for others to finish as well, which led to what the teachers liked to call attention-seeking behavior. It was easy to attribute to my home life; three brothers means I don't get as much attention as I did before they were born. I knew I wasn't exactly looking for attention, though. I just needed stimulation. I needed structure and challenging work to stay focused. It was the same story every grade. I liked to talk and disrupt class with friends; I got bored easily, and I couldn't focus. This was the theme of my academic life until I was 16.

When I was in my junior year of high school, I went to the doctor and opened up about some of my difficulties in class. I hadn't thought that I had ADHD before, probably because I didn't really know much about it. I went to a psychiatrist referred by my doctor and took a two-hour test that indicated that I had ADHD. It was an interesting time, and I remember feeling relieved that I wasn't just a "bad" kid or dumb. I also worried about the stigma and what people would think about me. I had a lot of conflicting emotions that I struggled to process at the time.

I started on medication and worked with the psychiatrist on organizational skills and better habits. I knew the medication was a tool, not the solution, so I wanted to develop ways to manage my ADHD without relying too much on medication. I didn't know at the time that this would be a long journey of testing strategies and tactics to build positive habits in my life. I didn't know how frustrating ADHD can be at times, especially as an adult.

Since college, I've balanced three attitudes related to my ADHD. I can be optimistic and motivated to work on myself, put effort into my habits and structure, and feel I have a good solution since I know the problem. I battle with feelings of hopelessness and frustration when I realize that this is a lifelong process. I used to feel like it was me versus ADHD, but now I know it's me versus myself. I stopped trying to fight against my "ADHD brain" and developed a set of compromises and tricks to be successful. My therapist doesn't like when I say I "trick my brain" into doing something, but that's the best way to describe it.

You didn't come here to read about my life story, but I hope you've been able to see a bit of yourself and your own struggles in my story. In the next few sections, I'll break down what has worked for me, what works now, and what hasn't worked. Before we jump into that, I want to stress the importance of failure. I used to be extremely afraid of failure and chose not to do certain things or take risks because of this fear. I've since realized that failure is how we grow. It's how we learn what *not* to do, and it gets us closer to knowing what we need to do to succeed. Embrace failure and defeat in your own life and use it as a lesson. It shouldn't prevent you from doing something, it should make you want it even more. You only have to get it right

once to see results.

Mixing Business With Pleasure

It's probably not specific to people with ADHD, but I hate mundane tasks. There's nothing worse to me than folding laundry, sweeping, or working on an Excel sheet all day. You may have heard about getting into a "flow state," where you're completely focused on a task or activity without thoughts about yourself or even your performance. People without ADHD, or neurotypical people, can easily slip into and out of the flow state to complete these mundane tasks and activities.

I didn't even know what the flow state felt like until I got on medication for ADHD. As I mentioned in the first section, medication is just a tool in your ADHD toolbox, but it's a game-changer for the mundane. Unfortunately, you won't be on medication 100% of the time. I've found that the best way to get through mundane tasks is to establish a reward that is tangible and immediate once the task is done. You probably don't feel more motivated to sweep the floor because it'll contribute to a cleaner house. That's the unfortunate truth.

I had friends growing up who would get money for a good report card. While my parents didn't do anything like this, and good grades were expected, I suspect that this reward structure wouldn't have made much of a difference. $100 in three months has little to no bearing on my motivation to do well on a test tomorrow. My dad used to take me to get a milkshake or a burger the day I took a test. It didn't matter if I did well or not; we would go and get a shake. I realized later that I still did want to do well on the tests because I worried that my dad would stop this tradition if I didn't do well. I also didn't want to let him down.

You probably *want* a cleaner house, but it's difficult to connect that with sweeping the floor. Instead, try putting the task before the reward. If you're into video games, you can tell yourself that sweeping the floor for half an hour means you can play your favorite game as soon as you're done. The reward can be as small as a snack or watching a TV show, but it is important to connect the two together. Establish tangible rewards and you'll develop an almost Pavlovian response to some of your most boring tasks and activities, turning them into good habits.

Doing It for Five Minutes

Another way I like to "trick my brain" is the five-minute rule. It's a combination of two helpful motivators. The first trick is if it takes less than five minutes, just do it now. Bed needs to be made? It'll take two minutes; get it done. The second trick is convincing yourself to do something for five minutes. Starting a new project at work or a school paper that seems daunting? Do it for five minutes, then let yourself take a break. I promise you won't want that break after five minutes.

This tactic is another way to build a foundation of stronger habits in your daily life. I struggle to find the motivation to do things, and as I get older, I also struggle with finding the energy to do things. This creates a mental barrier between me and the task at hand, and it's a tough negative thought loop to break.

ADHD and Relationships

This can be a big one. I could talk about ADHD and relationships all day. It's a complex subject, and as I mentioned earlier, ADHD is unique to each individual. When I see someone frequently, like at work or when I was in school, I can have a solid, normal relationship with them. However, if someone moves away or a pandemic happens, it's very easy for me to forget to reach out. It becomes harder to remember commitments, communicate, and nurture that relationship.

Another factor that plays a role in relationships is the inattentiveness and focus issues. I've often been told I don't have a filter, and I do tend to say what comes to mind. It's something I've worked at enough to where I don't get myself into trouble, but unless I'm consciously aware of it, it's easy to interrupt someone when they're speaking or tune them out. It isn't because I want to be rude or don't care what the person has to say, but I know that if I don't blurt out what I want to say at that exact moment, I'll lose my train of thought and look like an idiot in my response.

Active listening can be hard for those with ADHD. We can latch on to something seemingly insignificant and tune out the rest of what someone is saying, or we might think of something completely unrelated while trying to stay engaged. It's as frustrating for us as it is for the individual with whom we're engaging. With enough practice, the proper medication, and mindfulness, it does get easier. I can have an extensive, thought-provoking conversation with a friend and stay engaged, or speak with my boss for an hour about a project and stay on track the whole time.

Romantic relationships can similarly be a struggle. Everything I mentioned in this section applies to these relationships, along with another set of challenges that can cause friction. Many with ADHD tend to make impulsive financial decisions, which can strain their relationship with their significant other. Tackling impulsivity and communication challenges early on is important, and establishing boundaries and setting times to talk about and review finances can be very beneficial.

I can't stress the importance of communication in your relationships. It's important for *anyone* in a relationship to communicate, but even more so for someone with ADHD. It's almost like speaking to someone in a different language, and communication is your translator. Overthinking is another feature of ADHD, so you can easily convince yourself of the worst possible scenario and let it fester if you're not careful.

Commitments tend to be difficult, too. I always arrive early, whether for work, a date, or an appointment, due to my fear of being late and being labeled as someone who's always late. This isn't the case for many people with ADHD, and it's not because they don't care or don't value their commitments, it's just simply hard to keep track of. Time is weird for people with ADHD. We live very much in the present and struggle to plan for the future. If I have a doctor's appointment at 3 PM, I'll spend all day thinking about it, how I need to get there on time, and I won't relax until I'm there on time.

Workplace Strategies

Navigating the workplace with ADHD can present its challenges, but with the right strategies, you can thrive professionally. First, you need to understand your own ADHD patterns and how they affect your work. This self-awareness will be the foundation for your success. One of the most effective strategies is to create a structured daily routine. I like to set clear daily goals and prioritize tasks. Tools like to-do lists, digital calendars, and reminder apps can be your best friends in keeping you on track. I find that breaking down complex tasks into smaller, manageable steps can make your workload feel less overwhelming, too.

Time management is another key aspect. I recommend using techniques like the Pomodoro Technique, which involves working for short, focused intervals followed by breaks, to maintain productivity without feeling burnt out. It's all about finding a rhythm that suits your attention span.

In meetings or when receiving instructions, don't hesitate to ask for clarification if needed. It's perfectly okay to seek extra information to ensure you fully understand your tasks and responsibilities. The fear of looking dumb is always outweighed by doing something wrong and looking like you don't know what you're doing. I can listen to someone giving me instructions and within a minute forget half of what they said. I know that I need to take notes to ensure I get all of the necessary information. Most people won't have any issues if you ask for further clarification or take notes while they speak.

Minimizing distractions is essential. Create a clutter-free workspace and consider noise-canceling headphones if your workplace is noisy. Block distracting websites or apps during work hours to stay focused. I clean off my desk at the end of each workday, making sure I don't have any loose paper, books, or clutter for the next day. It's also a great way to separate your workday from your evenings, especially if you work from home. If your job allows it, taking breaks to go for a walk can be very beneficial. I have one call that I take while walking every day, and it helps break the day up and makes the conversation more casual and creative.

Letting your employer know you have ADHD is typically recommended, but I have my reservations depending on the company. It can be used against you, even if it shouldn't be, legally. I avoid letting my employers know for the most part since there is usually a stigma and could impact your growth at the company. You should let your HR department know when you start, but I don't typically recommend sharing with coworkers or your boss.

ADHD and Self-Esteem

Living with ADHD can bring unique emotional challenges, and many with ADHD struggle with self-esteem. It's not uncommon to feel frustrated, overwhelmed, or even defeated by the daily struggles that ADHD can present. However, you should remember that ADHD is just one aspect of who you are, and it doesn't define your worth. Self-acceptance is key. Embrace your ADHD as a part of your identity rather than a flaw. Understand that it comes with strengths like creativity, spontaneity, and hyperfocus. Celebrating and acknowledging these positives can boost your self-esteem.

Setting realistic goals is another important step for self-esteem and confidence. Break down your objectives into manageable tasks and celebrate each achievement, no matter how small. This not only builds confidence but also provides a sense of accomplishment. Seeking support from loved ones can be immensely beneficial, too. Share your challenges and triumphs with them. Their encouragement and understanding can provide a much-needed emotional boost.

Mindfulness and meditation are important in one's journey when dealing with ADHD. Just a few minutes a day in the morning can get you in the right mindset to tackle the day. There are plenty of free apps that will guide you through a short meditation session that helps quiet and calm your mind, reduce anxiety and stress, and put you in a good mood. Since starting this, I have seen amazing benefits in various aspects of my life.

Therapy is another tool that I can't recommend enough. Many feel like a burden when speaking to friends and family about their challenges and thoughts, so take advantage of this outlet and express yourself freely with a professional. You'll find more tools and insight when speaking with someone who knows what you're dealing with daily. I go to therapy once or twice a month and feel much lighter afterward. It is important to find the right therapist, however. I recommend shopping around and finding someone who understands your struggles and challenges.

Remember that self-esteem is an ongoing journey. Be patient with yourself and practice self-compassion. Understand that setbacks are a part of life, and they don't diminish your worth. Over time, as you learn to embrace your uniqueness and build on your strengths, you'll find that self-confidence and self-acceptance can flourish, allowing you to thrive personally and professionally.

Nutrition and Exercise

Nutrition plays a crucial role in managing ADHD. While there's not a specific ADHD diet, some dietary choices can make a positive impact. You can start by incorporating a balanced diet rich in whole grains, lean protein, fruits, and vegetables. These foods provide a steady supply of energy and essential nutrients, helping to stabilize mood and improve focus. Omega-3 fatty acids found in fatty fish like salmon, walnuts, and flaxseeds are known to support brain health. They can enhance cognitive function and might help with ADHD symptoms. Additionally, reducing or eliminating artificial additives and preservatives, which can exacerbate ADHD symptoms in some individuals, is important when deciding what to eat.

Exercise is another fantastic tool in managing ADHD. Physical activity has been shown to boost the release of dopamine and norepinephrine, neurotransmitters that play a role in attention and focus. Regular exercise can help reduce impulsivity and hyperactivity, common traits of ADHD. You don't have to spend hours in the gym daily to see results, start with a short walk or bike ride and make it a routine. Find an activity you enjoy, as consistency is key. Make it a habit to experience long-term benefits. Moreover, exercise contributes to better sleep quality, which is crucial for managing ADHD. It helps regulate your circadian rhythm and ensures you wake up refreshed and ready to tackle the day.

Coping Mechanisms

I've put together a list of coping mechanisms that should help you find effective ways to navigate some of ADHD's unique challenges. Some of these are mentioned already, and some may be new.

1. **Time Management:** Time can slip away when you have ADHD, but techniques like using calendars, alarms, or time-blocking can help you stay organized and meet deadlines.

2. **Task Prioritization:** Break tasks into smaller, manageable parts and prioritize them. Tackling one thing at a time can prevent feeling overwhelmed.

3. **Mindfulness and Meditation:** Practicing mindfulness can enhance focus and reduce impulsivity. Short meditation sessions can be incredibly beneficial.

4. **Healthy Lifestyle Choices:** Regular exercise, a balanced diet, and quality sleep are essential. They can improve your mood, increase energy levels, and aid concentration.

5. **Medication:** Consult a healthcare professional about medication options. They can be a valuable tool in managing ADHD symptoms.

6. **Structured Environment:** Create a clutter-free and organized workspace. Structure can minimize distractions and boost productivity.

7. **Support Network:** Build a support system of friends, family, or support groups who understand ADHD and can provide encouragement and understanding.

8. **Therapy and Counseling:** Behavioral therapy can equip you with practical strategies for managing symptoms and addressing challenges in relationships and work.

9. **Self-Awareness:** Understand your strengths and weaknesses. Knowing how ADHD affects you personally can guide your coping strategies.

10. **Stress Management:** Adopt stress-reduction techniques like deep breathing, progressive muscle relaxation, or hobbies you enjoy.

11. **Flexibility:** Be kind to yourself. Understand that setbacks happen, and flexibility is crucial in adapting to changing circumstances.

Coping mechanisms are highly individualized. What works best for one person may differ for another. Experiment and find the combination of strategies that fits you best. You should also understand that this is a lifelong process, meaning your mechanisms may evolve or change over time.

Practical Exercises

Like the coping mechanisms mentioned in the previous section, you can implement practical exercises into your daily life to see results. Important exercises include time management techniques, journaling, visualization, self-reflection, goal-setting, and planning. Try implementing one or two of these at a time and find what works for you.

Time management, as mentioned a few times in this eBook, is important for those with ADHD. I have found success using the Pomodoro method, and there are free apps that you can download to try this method. It helps me because it breaks larger tasks into bite-sized pieces that show me my progress and lets me take breaks without feeling guilty.

Journaling is a fantastic exercise to add to your routine. I journal when I'm stressed, upset, or need to put my thoughts into words to make sense of something. It feels like therapy, leaving me feeling lighter and more confident in myself afterward. I tend to use the Notes app on my phone, but you may prefer pen and paper. It helps to look back on your past journals, too. You'll see how far you've come and reflect on your mindset when you journal frequently.

You can use visualization techniques to picture yourself successfully completing tasks or achieving goals. Visualization can boost motivation and increase confidence, and it makes things feel less intense or unachievable. If you have a job interview coming up, visualize the conversation going well. Imagine how you'll respond to certain questions, how you'll feel when you get an offer, and picture yourself in the role. It helps make the intangible feel tangible.

Self-reflection can sometimes be a combination of journaling and visualization. Ask yourself how you felt in a certain situation, what made you feel how you did, and areas in which you can improve. Be kind to yourself when reflecting, as it can be easy to beat yourself up if you're not careful. During self-reflection, you can set goals and plan for the future, too. Develop a list of things you need to do to achieve success. Visualize yourself achieving that success and putting in the work to get to the finish line.

Conclusion

I hope you found this eBook beneficial, or at least informative. Everyone deals with ADHD differently, which makes it a unique topic to attempt to write about. I'm not perfect, and I certainly haven't mastered my ADHD, but I've accepted that I may never fully "overcome" this condition. ADHD will be a part of me until the day I die, for better or for worse. It took me a long time to accept that. I'm frequently jealous of more neurotypical people, like my brothers, because things come easily to them that I have to spend a long time working at. But other things come easily to me because I can look at a problem differently.

I wouldn't go as far as saying ADHD is a superpower like many do these days, but it's not all bad. I can hyperfocus on a subject and get an enormous amount of work done in a short period of time. The downside is that I'm always seeking something new that interests me. My hobbies and interests are always changing, and something I may have been obsessed with a month ago is boring today. This becomes a problem when it's an expensive hobby, but since I've been able to identify my everchanging interests, I've been able to better manage my spending.

The best thing you can do is accept the challenges that come with ADHD and learn to live with them. You can't completely eradicate them and you can't ignore them, so you're left with one option. The need for constant stimulation can easily lead to depression and anxiety, so implementing structure in your life is imperative. Think back to the times in your life when you were the happiest and try to replicate that structure. Keep notes of the ways in which you develop habits and a routine so if you ever regress, you'll have a guide to help you get back to where you were at.

I'd like to speak a little about addiction before I wrap this up. Addiction goes hand in hand with our constant need for stimulation, which can take over if you're not careful. You can be addicted to something as simple as a mobile game on your phone. Anything that can stimulate or appease your brain's reward center should be carefully monitored and done in moderation. Many with ADHD suffer from drug addiction. It's an easy route to take and an extremely hard hole to dig yourself out of. Seek professional help as early as possible if you notice yourself becoming addicted to something unhealthy for you and try to replace the habit with a more positive one, like going to the gym or cooking.